Boost your Fat away Detox

BOOST YOUR BODY IN 7 DAYS TO A HEALTHY LEVEL

Healthy Clean Body

ByRenee Anderson

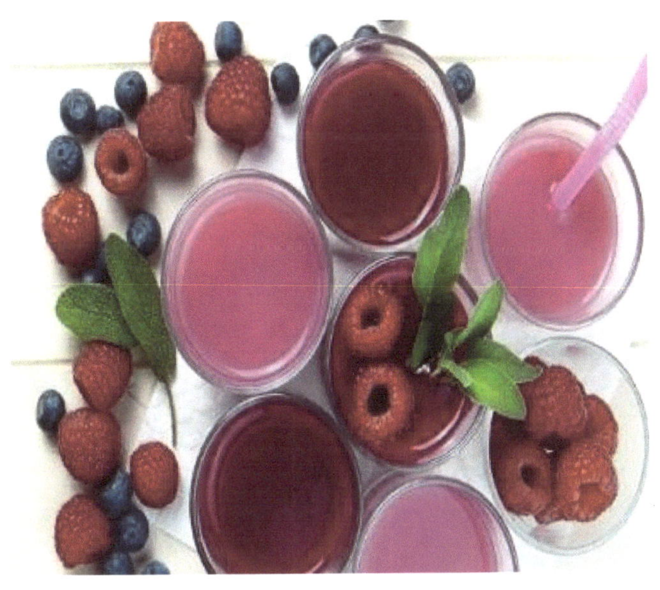

Boost your Fat away Detox
7 Days

Content

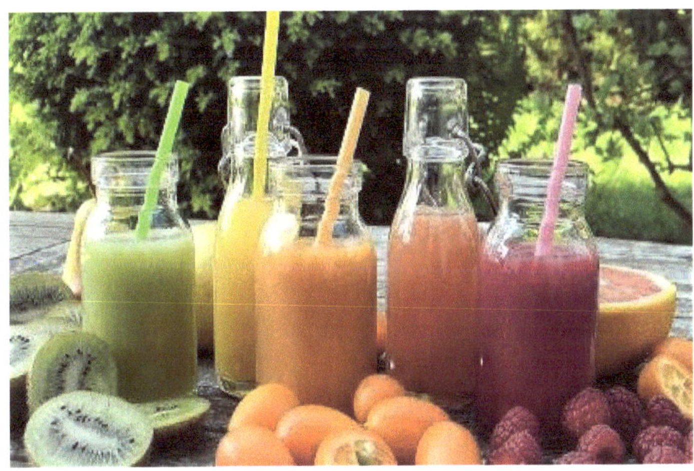

Introduction

And here you have arrived, you are planning to give your body a healthy boost, clean sitter, all the waste and toxins and free radicals, a push in the back to tackle the extra pounds and adopt a healthy lifestyle and get rid of Fat. You have made a very good choice, one of the best investments you will make in your life namely in your own body and health.

In my opinion, a better investment is not there because your body and health have to last for years and if we do this the right way you will have the most valuable reward you will ever get life.

By starting with the Boost your Fat away Detox, you start a healthy journey to a healthy cleaned body.

At the end of the ride, you will have cleaned your body from various waste and toxins, a number of pounds lighter (for each different but at least 2 kilos) and feel good about yourself.

And most importantly you will have given your body the delicious treatment it deserves.

You will feel Great!!

Let's Get Started.

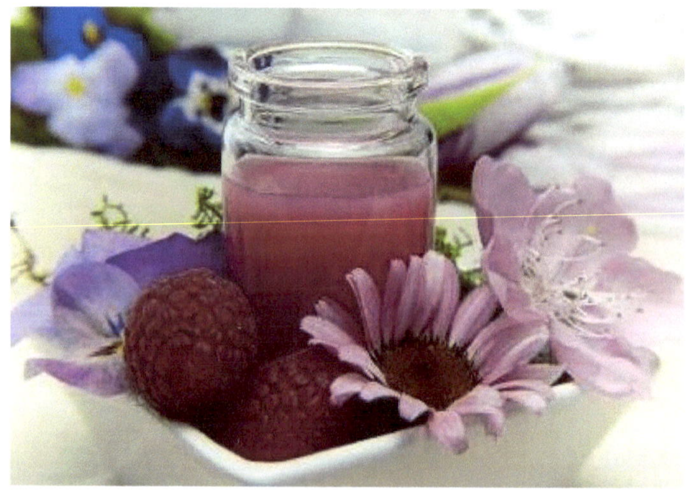

What is Detox?

First, let's go deeper into the question of what IS DETOX?

Detox is a word that we have borrowed from English Grammar with the meaning of "detoxification". Everyone knows there's only one way to detox your body or detoxify it: Stop consuming things that are toxic and unhealthy for your body, bad habits like drugs, alcohol but also and what I'm talking about food.
You must stop taking what your body just doesn't respond to properly. But we all know that this is certainly difficult in this time of quick bites, stress and crowds.
Difficult if you're not used to it but certainly not impossible and with the JUICE DETOX 7 DAYS you're already on the right track.

So, when we talk about a Detox, we'll have a program of a few days to get rid of toxins released by nutrition, stress etc. in our bodies and clean waste in our bodies.

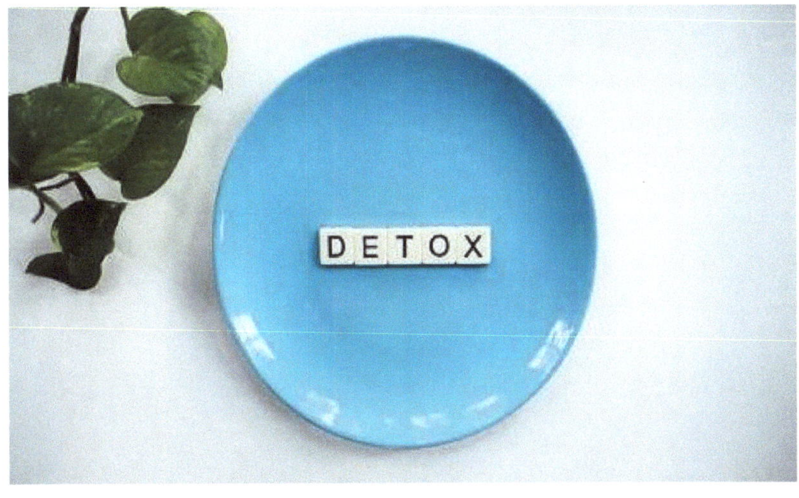

Why is a Detox good for our bodies?

There are a number of reasons why a Detox cure is good for our bodies, of course there are proponents and opponents for this, but I am certainly a supporter of that for the following reasons.

I find this for both men and women among us and if you are 40+ then it certainly has its advantages.

* Kick Start to lose a number of pounds. And if you had already started losing weight and standing still (this happens after a while), a DETOX gives you just that extra push in the back to move the scales. You will be eating these 7 days a lot less, healthier and you clean your body at the same time.

*You're losing weight.

* By keeping the schedule these 7 days and not taking other "bad" fats, sugars, unhealthy foods we purify our bodies of waste and free radicals, our skin is going to look cleaner and better and our cells refreshed.

* We're going to sleep better, because you get less to no caffeine or bad sugars, you sleep better.

* You get more energy, through all the healthy juices and smoothies you get in, you also get a lot more minerals and vitamins inside.
Even if you eat less you will feel much more energetic.

* After your 40th life year your body changes in various ways, your body also acidified much faster so that a lot of waste is released and we need to make a little more effort to clean our bodies, A Detox certainly helps you get rid from this waste faster.

The advantages in a row.

The advantages are certainly to be found as I described before.

You're losing weight.

You're getting rid of your body from waste.

You're getting more energy.

You get better skin.

You give yourself a start on a healthier lifestyle.

You're becoming more aware of what you take in to your body.

You'll experience a better night's sleep.

When you shouldn't start a detox is:

If you are Pregnant.

When you're taking medication.

Chest feeding babies.

Have an eating disorder.

Whether another medical condition or complaint

I really advise everyone to consult your own doctor first if in doubt.

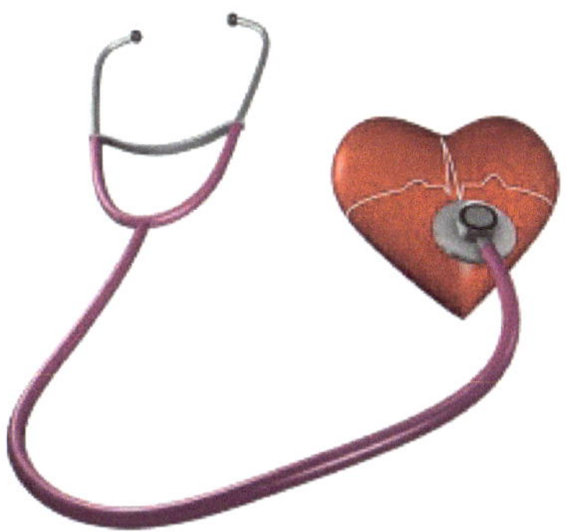

Starting the Boost your Fat away DETOX 7 Days

If you start the Boost Your Fat Away DETOX 7 Days and you've never followed a detox before, I recommend you to start reducing food 2 days in advance before you start. These two days you're probably going to phase out your daily intake of food.

And get used to drinking as much water as possible (min. 2 liters of water per day).

Try to leave these products behind these two dismantling days.

Coffee Sugar

Packaged foods like Cookies, chips etc. actually everything that is in a bag or plastic.

Alcohol (all types)

Meat

For the Die Harts among us who have done this several times, I recommend this and otherwise start nicely at day 1.

During detoxing you can get certain side effects but this doesn't have to be for everyone. If you do experience them, you know it could be because of the detoxing.

Side effects

*pimples (this is because the waste is removed from your body but they will go away)

*Bad breath (brush your mouth for fresh breath more often)

*Headache (your body needs to get used to withdrawal of caffeine)

*Nausea (your body needs to adapt)

During the Boost Your Fat Away DETOX 7 DAYS drink at least 2 liters of water to clean your body. ***Tip: Put lemon juice in it, contains vitamin C and has a cleansing effect.***

Well if you are ready to start the Juice Detox 7 Days and you made all your precautions the days before, I will now tell you how it is going to work these 7 days.

Juice Detox diet consists of drinking juices and smoothies that consist of many vegetables and fruit. You don't eat nothing else these 7 days. With this Juice Detox, the construction and dismantling are incredibly important. It is not good for your body to stop eating immediately that's why I recommend the 2 days advance withdrawal to get used to the diet. Neither is it good for you to immediately eat a hot meal right after the seventh day you have to build it up again. This type of detoxing, you can do it for example, once every six months or once a year.

The things that you can do while you are detoxing these 7 days to promote the blood circulation and to dispose the waste that is coming out of your system is

Ensuring good blood flow during the detox: You can do this by taking a cold shower, among other things. Start and end your shower with a cold shower for a minute and you optimally stimulate your blood flow.

Disposing waste out of your system: Go to the sauna regularly. By sweating you remove a lot of waste and you clean your body that way. Your Skin will look and feel soft again and your pores will be fresh and open again A good scrub will help you feel clean and fit after you get out of the sauna.

Sports and yoga are always good for the human body. Sweating, a high heart rate and deep breathing improve the detoxification effect in your body. Try to get every day exercise it does not have to be long or for hours try between 10 30 minutes a day. But don't exaggerate. Exercising too intensively is not good during your juice detox because you will burn to much calories and it will drain you from your energy that will need.

Go outside for walks these 7 days and take the time for meditation.

Good breathing brings fresh oxygen into your body that ensures a better lymphatic system.

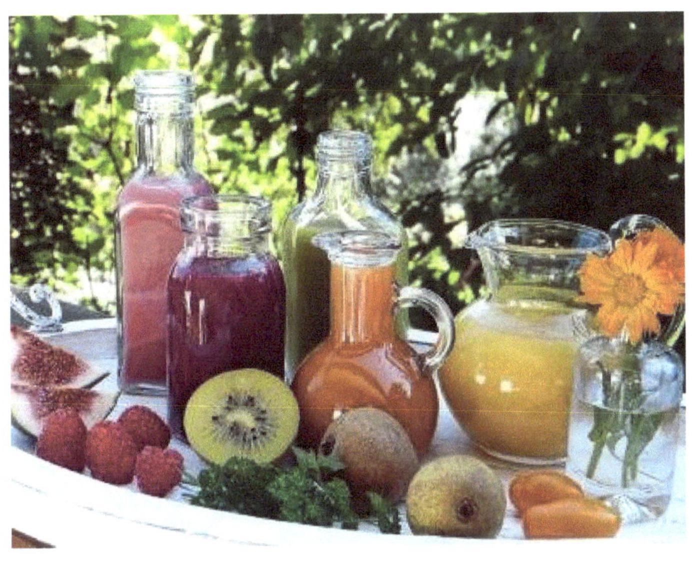

The Boost your Fat away Detox 7 Days

Through out this book you will find the most healthys and delicouse detox shakes, smooties with all ther ingredients and how to make them. You will allso find the benefits of the urbs and fruits that are in the detox shakes and smoothies. So enjoy them all and see what the delicious shakes can do for you in just 7 days.

Replace all your meals that you have in a normal day with one of the smoothies and juices in this book. Make sure that you have at **least 4** of them a day and that you drink a lot of water. Try to use the organic products because they are not processed and are better for your body.

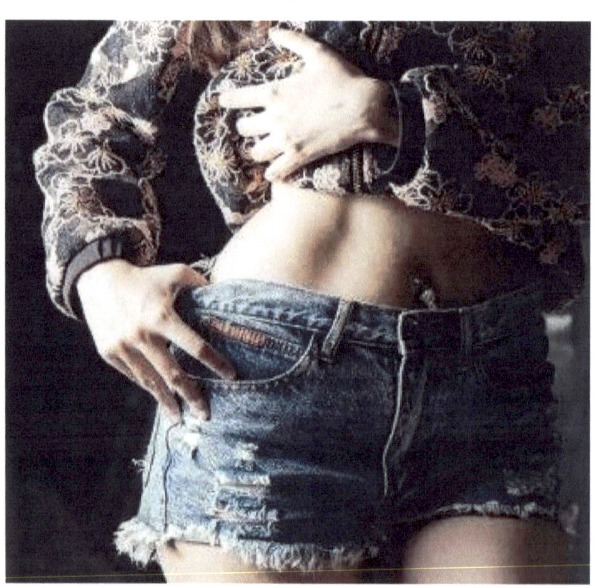

Apple / Beet Juice

- 1 apple
- 1 lemon
- 1 peeled beet
- 1 bunch (say 5 stalks) coriander
- 3 stalks of celery
- 200 ml coconut milk/water try to get the organic.
- a slice of ginger root (peel it)

Blend this all together in a blender.

Beets are great for cleansing your liver and supporting your blood. Beets contain a lot of iron so we won't juice them more than 2 times a week. Apples are excellent in the overall cleaning of your body. An apple contains vitamins B1, B2, B6, C and E. It also offers a variety of sugars such as dextrose, fructose and sucrose but the healthy ones. The combination of acids in the apple is responsible for the taste. In addition, it contains a number of minerals, such as calcium, magnesium and potassium, as well as pectin and fibers. About 85 percent of the apple consists of water

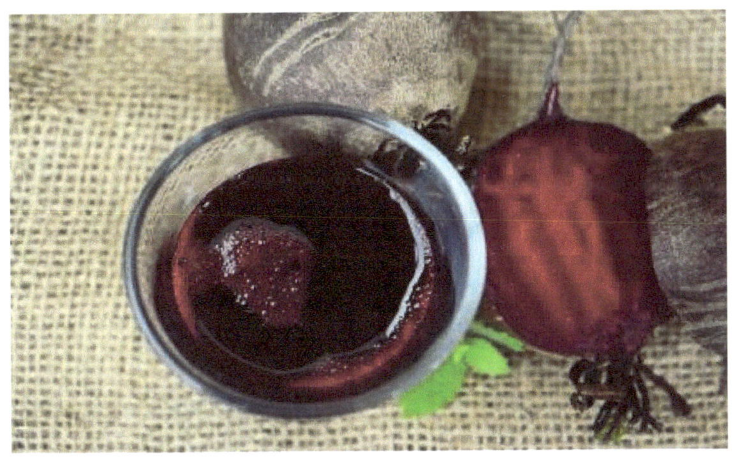

Basil and peach-detox Smoothie

- 7/9 basil leaves
- 4 peaches
- 1 glass of cold water

1. You need a blender or a food processor
2. Coarsely chop the peaches and mix them with a food processor.
3. Add the Basil leaves and the Glass of water
3. Pour the peach smoothie into a glass.
5. Stir well.

Benefits of basil and peaches:

Basil helps to lower cholesterol, regulates blood sugar levels and has antimicrobial and anti-inflammatory character traits.
Peaches are a good source of various minerals, including:
Magnesium: Magnesium affects many body processes. Among other things, it contributes to strong bones, a healthy heart and vascular system, the reduction of insulin resistance and a healthy energy level.
Zinc: Zinc is important for our metabolism, our immune system, our brains and for keeping our skin, eyes and hair healthy.
Iron: We need iron for the production of red blood cells and therefore also for a healthy energy level and the prevention of anemia.
Calcium: Calcium is mainly known for contributing to healthy bones, but it is also important for the absorption and transport of other minerals and for the proper functioning of our nerves and muscles.
Potassium: Potassium helps to keep your blood pressure healthy, reducing your risk of cardiovascular disease. Furthermore, potassium contributes to the prevention of fluid retention and kidney stones. Peaches also help to mobilize fat.

Resistance Smoothie

- 50gr. Spinach
- 2/4 cucumber
- 1/2 lemon
- 3 apples
- 2/4 pineapple
- 1/2 avocado
- 1 glass water

Blend this all together in a food processor

This shake stimulates your resistance system, it is rich in potassium, vitamin C and iron. The folic acid in avocado supports the production of various important hormones, such as serotonin, dopamine and norepinephrine. These hormones have an effect on our human body Energy balance Appetite night's sleep.
Avocado has a positive effect on the above points.

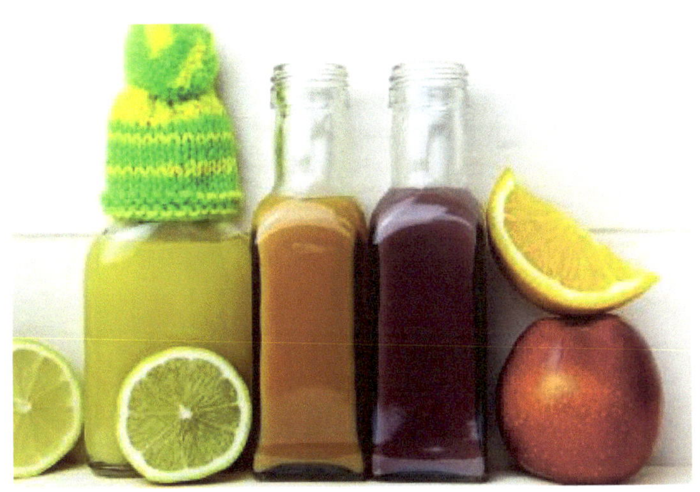

Boosting metabolism juice

- 10 strawberries
- 10 cranberries
- 10 blueberries
- half grapefruit
- a few mints leave

Blend this all together in a food processor

Benefits of Grapefruit, Cranberries and Blueberries:
Strawberries are rich in antioxidants. They help to regulate blood sugar levels and reduce the risk of cardiovascular disease. Grapefruit can help with weight loss. It contains various properties associated with weight loss, especially the fiber content, that help saturate and reduce calorie intake. In addition, grapefruit contains few calories but a lot of water, which can also contribute to weight loss.
Cranberries strengthen your immunity, have anti-inflammatory and antioxidant properties and protect against urinary tract infection.
Blueberries help maintain normal blood sugar levels, and improve brain function.
Antioxidants are important. They protect our bodies against free radical damage, unstable molecules that can damage the cell structure and that contribute to aging and diseases such as cancer. Blueberries are believed to contain the highest concentration of antioxidants of widely all of the consumed fruits and vegetables

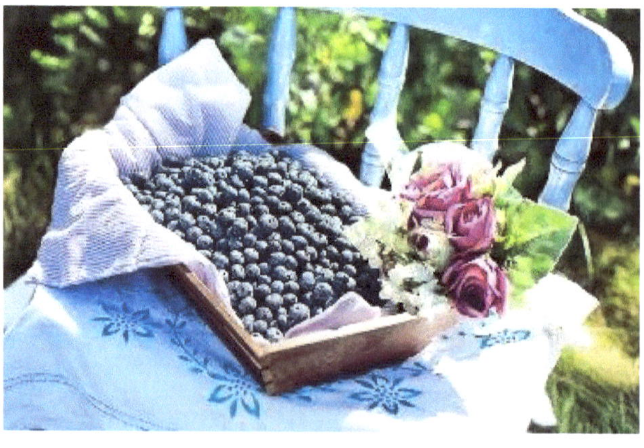

Ignition-free Smoothie

- 1 hand full of parsley
- 5 cm of peeled ginger root
- 1 lemon
- 1 cucumber (medium to small)
- 1 hand full coriander
- 150 ml of coconut water

Put the ingredients together with the coconut water in a food processor and blend it.

Benefits of Ginger and Parsley:
Ginger not only improves your digestion but is also a source of antioxidants. Parsley is moisture-repellent and provides fresh breath. It also stimulates digestion and is anti-inflammatory just like ginger.

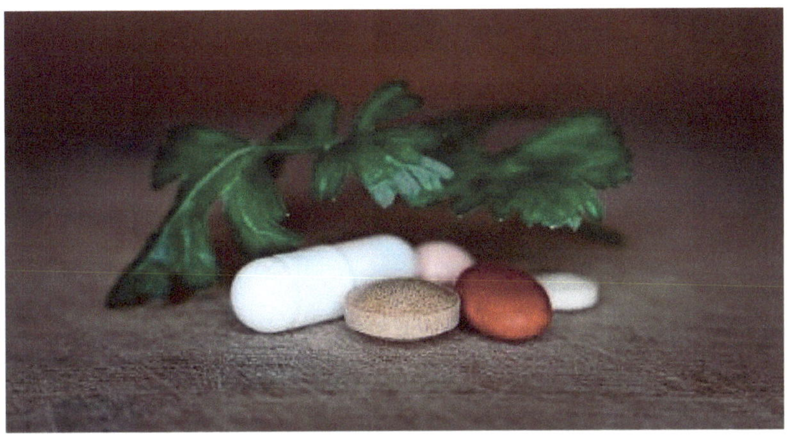

Carrot fat burner Smoothie

- 2 carrot
- 1 half a bunch of celery
- 1,5lime
- 1/2 teaspoon ground pepper

Put this together in a blender

Benefits of Carrots and Celery
Carrot juice is extremely useful for the prevention of cardiovascular disease. Carrots contain a lot of fiber. These fibers help your cholesterol levels, but also your intestines are very happy with these fibers. They help improve your intestinal flora, so that the good bacteria in your intestines are nourished and you are less likely to suffer from intestinal complaints. Fiber also ensures that you get a regular bowel movement and that you are saturated faster. Eating carrots also ensures that you feel full faster.
Celery is a food with negative calories and helps in burning calories. It also helps in lowering blood pressure.
Black pepper is rich in antioxidants and is an effective antimicrobial agent.
Lime is rich in vitamin C that is known to strengthen your immunity.

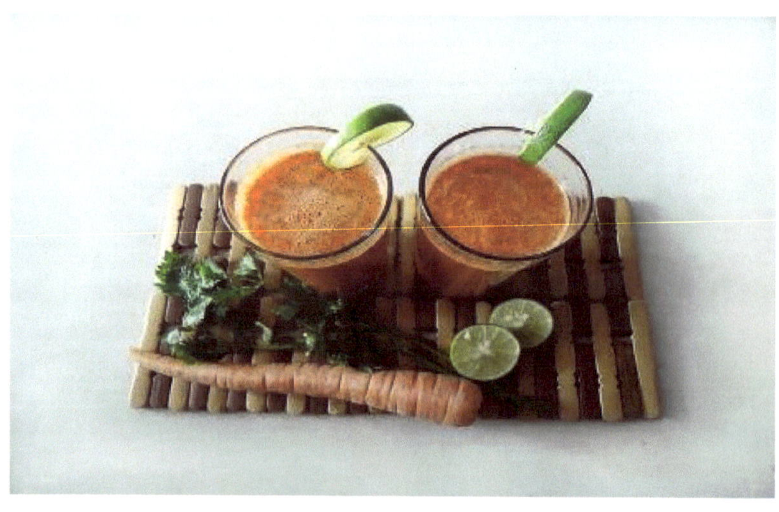

Good morning Smoothie

- 1 cup of coconut water
- 1 cup of raspberries
- 1 banana
- 1 cup of blueberries
- 1 table spoon of lemon juice
- 1 cup of ice cubes (less if you use frozen fruit!)

Place all the ingredients in the blender.
Do this in the order in which they appear in the list of ingredients., wait until everything is blend
The smoothie should trigger the detox process.
This means that this fiber-rich smoothie, with cleansing lemon, raspberries and blueberries, will help you detox by removing toxic substances from your body.

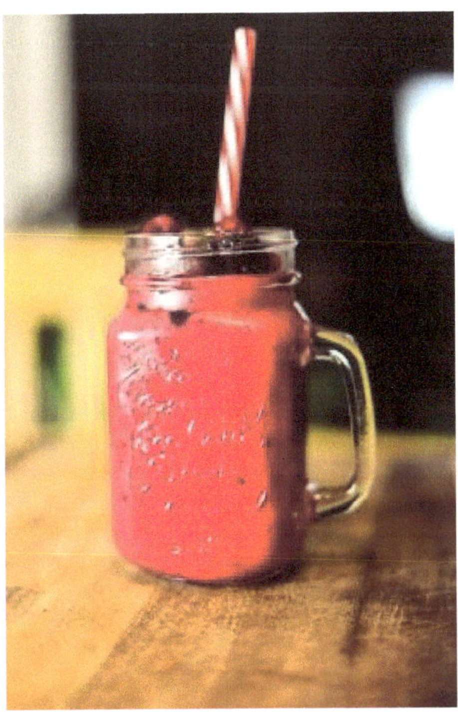

Deacidification Smoothie

- 1 bunch of celery
- 5 leaves of kale
- 1 green apple
- 3 branches fresh parsley
- 1 lime
- 1 lemon
- 5 cm of fresh ginger
- 1 cup of water

The basis of this detox juice is celery, a power in terms of nutritional value. It is particularly rich in potassium, folic acid, magnesium, calcium, iron, and essential amino acids. Moreover, celery is enormously deacidified, so it is actively helping deacidify your body.

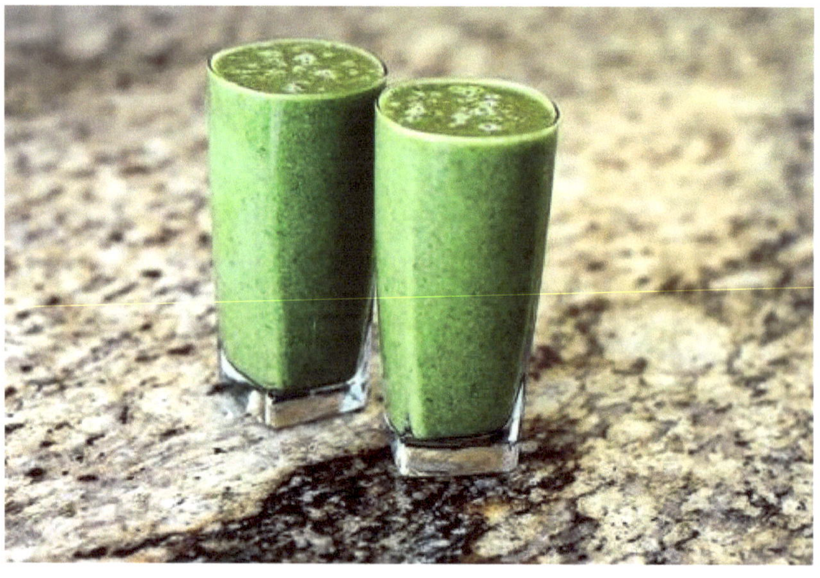

Cinnamon calorie burn Smoothie

- 1 cup of water
- 2 grapefruits
- 1 cinnamon stick /or half a tablespoon cinnamon powder
- ¼ teaspoon of salt

Blend this all together in a food processor or blender

Benefits:
Grapefruit and cinnamon help to reduce weight by improving insulin sensitivity.
Cinnamon has a regulating effect on blood sugar levels. It contributes to a slower absorption
of carbohydrates. Why is that important? If carbohydrates are slowly absorbed by the body,
your blood sugar levels show fewer spikes, which is better for your health. Your pancreas
needs to take action less often. Your appetite for snacks also decreases This is one of the
benefits of cinnamon.

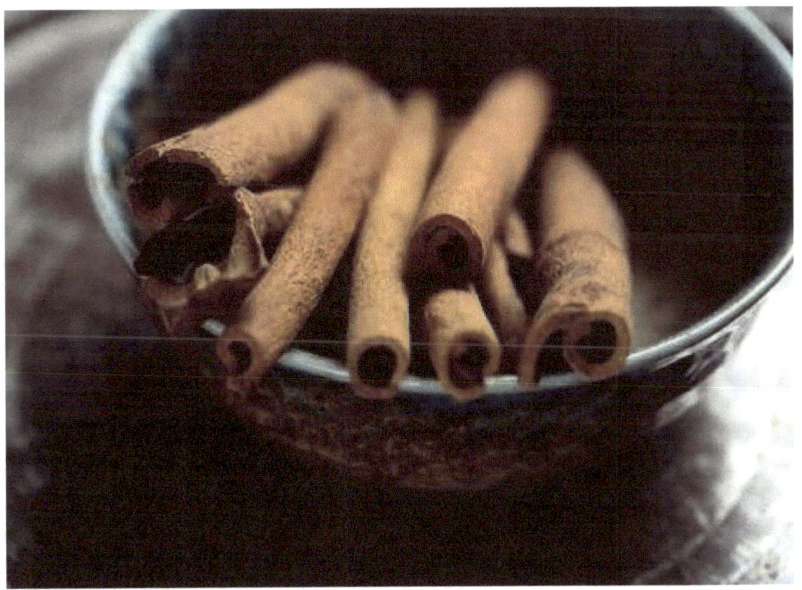

Mint Carrot Smoothie

- 4 carrots
- mint leaves of 4 branches
- 100ml orange juice (from fresh oranges)

Blend this together in a blender

Benefits:

This is not only a surprisingly tasty combination, but also incredibly effective: the beta-carotene in carrot is an excellent antioxidant. This juice helps to cleanse your liver, improves your digestion and helps lower your cholesterol. Oranges contain vitamin C, flavonoids and beta-carotene, which together act as a powerful antioxidant. This helps to cleanse your body and, if possible, can prevent cardiovascular diseases, degenerative diseases and cancer.

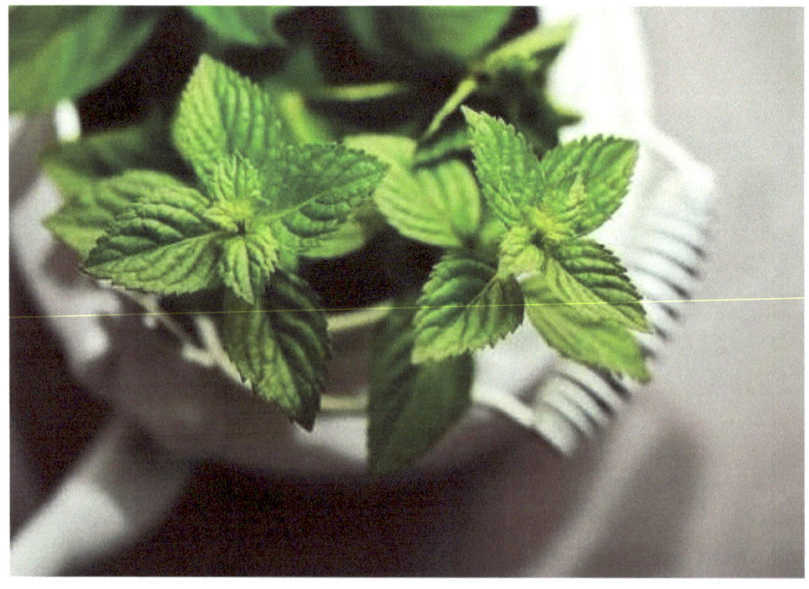

Fennel-cucumber Smoothie

- 1/2 fennel
- 1 cucumber
- 1 green apple
- 3 stalks of celery
- 1 cup of water/coconut water

Blend them all together in a blender.
If you don't have a Blender who can chop? Then chop the ingredients first and put it than in the blender.

Benefits:
This smoothie mix of fennel, cucumber, apple and celery. All four ingredients are full of nutrients that help digestion and also the metabolism. It keeps your hunger under control, drains excessive fluids out of your body and relieves inflammation caused by fluid retention.

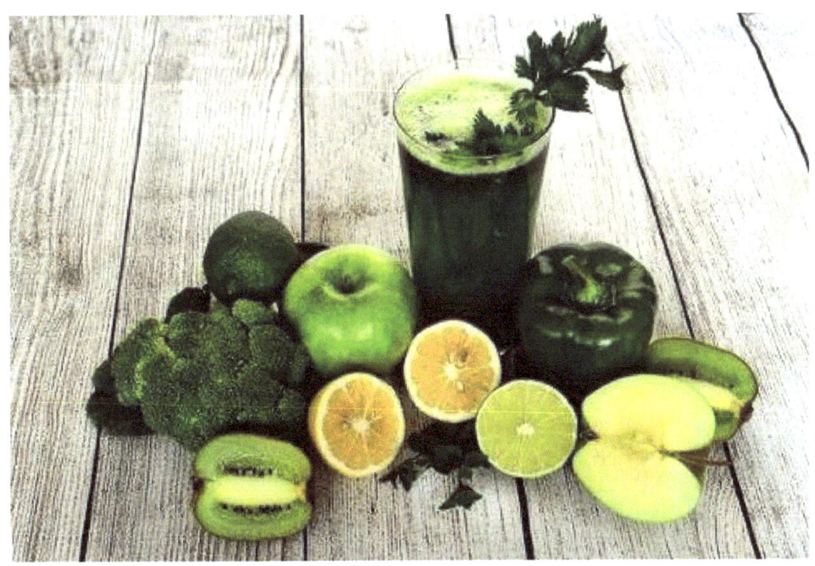

Vitamins Avocado Smoothie

- 1 avocado
- 1 banana
- 1/3 mango
- 1 peach
- 1 cup of orange juice or juice of 2 oranges (fresh)
- 2 table spoon of chia seed

Blend this all together in a blender, if you feel like the smoothie is to thick than ad some water to it.

Benefits:
Avocado increases the resistance, is full of fibers, minerals and vitamins, rich in Omega-3 and also healthy for your hair, skin and bones. Avocados are very nutritious and contain a wide variety of nutrients, including 20 different vitamins and minerals. Vitamin K, Vitamin E, Folic acid, Vitamin C, Potassium
Vitamin B5, Vitamin B6, amounts of magnesium, manganese, copper, iron, zinc, phosphorus, vitamin A, B1 (thiamin), B2 (riboflavin) and B3 (niacin).

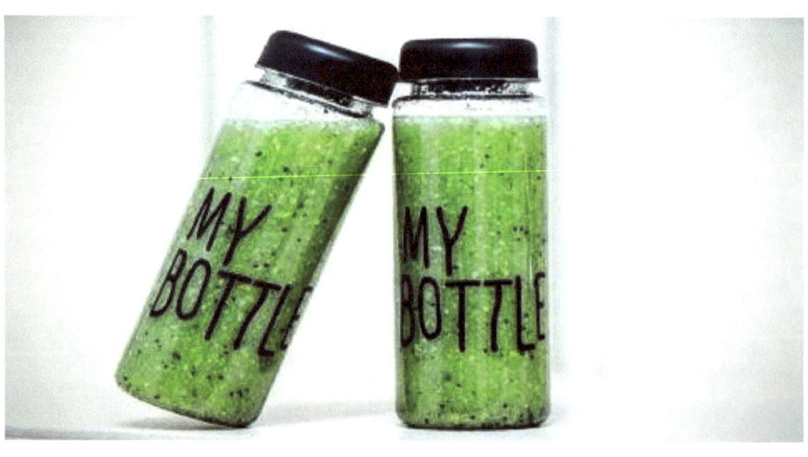

Sweet breakfast power Smoothie

- 4 dates
- 6 walnuts
- 5 hazelnuts
- 5 almonds
- ½ avocado
- 1 banana
- 2 tablespoons of cacao
- 1 cup of coconut milk (organic)
- 1 cup of ice

Blend this all together in a blender.
Benefits:
Avocado increases the resistance, is full of fibers, minerals and vitamins, rich in Omega-3. Almonds they contain high amount of calcium. They also contain a lot of fiber, vitamin E and magnesium. They help to lower cholesterol, reduce the risk of heart disease and protect against diabetes. Almonds contain a lot of proteins this is important if you exercise a lot or want to lose weight. Walnuts contain omega 3 fats, antioxidants and phytosterols. More than other nuts. Walnuts, would help prevent the risk of cancer and are healthy for your brain in case of complaints of depression. Walnuts also appear to prevent the risk of diseases, such as Alzheimer's. Hazelnuts are rich in unsaturated fats, magnesium, calcium and vitamins B and E. They also help reduce the risk of cancer. Bananas keep the digestive system healthy They provide stronger muscles. Thanks to the potassium content, eating bananas can help strengthen your muscles and at the same time promote recovery after a strong workout. They are good for blood pressure. Reduce the risk of cardiovascular disease. They are good for the skin.

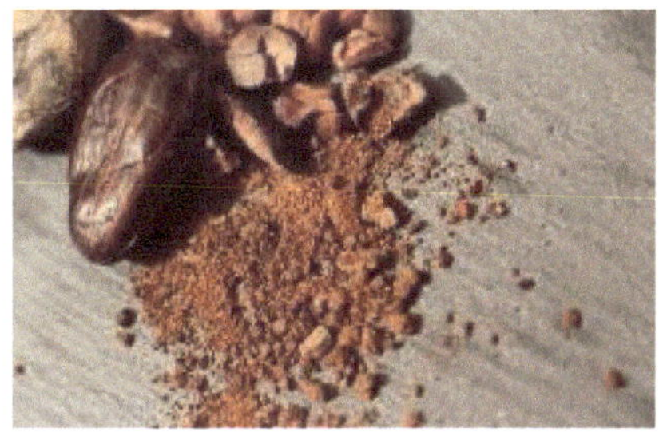

Pomegranate Smoothie

- 1 pomegranate
- 4 large strawberries (or 6 small ones)
- 6 pineapple cubes
- 1 banana
- 1/2 mango
- 1 cup of Almond Milk

Blend this all together in a blender

Benefits:
A pomegranate contains a high concentration of antioxidants. More than most other fruits. Antioxidants ensure that the risk of cancer is reduced. Pomegranate was compared with other components in an analysis. This showed that the juice of this fruit is the most effective in combating inflammation. It has an abundance of flavonoids. This in combination with the antibacterial property has proven to be very effective in removing bacteria that cause tooth decay and gum disease, so better for dental health. A pomegranate contains antioxidants. This ensures that the damage caused by the sun to our skin is limited by these antioxidants. They also counteract free radical and also stimulate the production of callogenesis

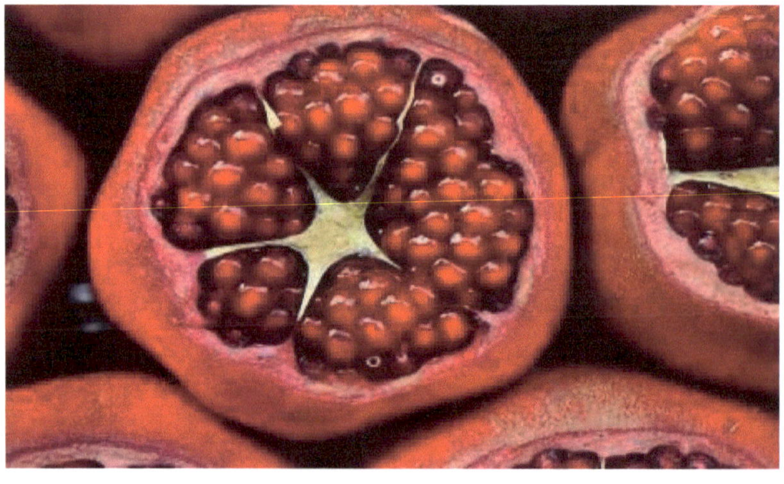

Kiwi Delight Smoothie

- 4 kiwis (green or gold)
- 1 banana
- 3 celery sticks
- 2 glasses of pineapple juice
- 1 mango
- 1 cup of ice

Blend everything together in a blender

Benefits:

Kiwis contain a lot of potassium, a mineral that ensures a proper fluid balance and a healthy blood pressure. A lot of foods have a high sodium content, so many people suffer from high blood pressure. Eating kiwis regularly can reduce this risk. Encourages weight loss. Kiwis are high in fiber. Correct PH value, Kiwis contain many minerals that ensure a healthy Ph value in your body. Healthy eyes, eating a kiwi every day,
reduces the chance of macular degeneration (also called retinal aging). Prevents fatigue.

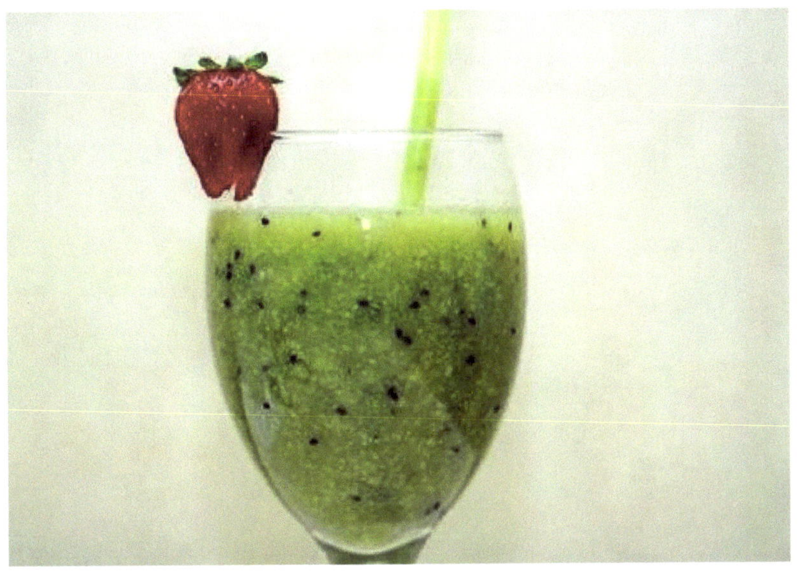

Not a Smoothie but good to have through the day

If you want to have a fit and healthy life style than you must introduce yourself with lemons on a daily bases and definitely start with it in the morning. Why? Well let me tell you why, before you think this is some kind non researched legend then think again.

Drinking lemon water every day is so healthy for your body and has many benefits. Toxins leave your body; Lemon water wakes up your organs in the morning. It moisturizes the lymphatic system and helps trigger digestion. You will go to the bathroom more often, because the water with lemon drives toxins out of your body. Citric acid also ensures proper functioning of the liver your liver will function better to get rid of toxins. Lemons have a high level of Vitamin C, your immune system will function better so your body can handle better viruses. The vitamin C is a stimulation for your brain and keeps blood sugar levels stable. The pectin in lemon juice reduces a feeling of hunger. Lemon water not only helps with weight loss, but also prevents bad skin, wrinkles and skin spots and detoxifies your body, it can achieve by containing a large number (antioxidant) substances to help inhibit cancer.

So why not start the day with fresh lemon water and throughout the day.

Our body would welcome it.

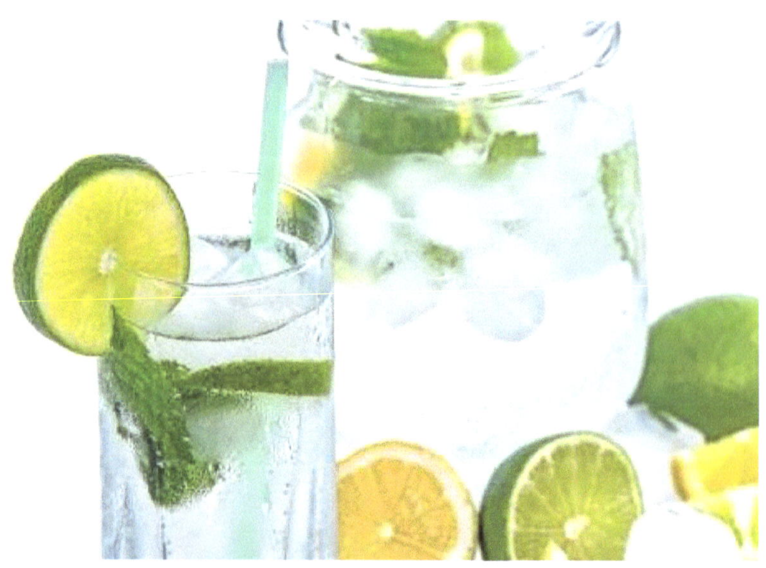

Spinach Smoothie with a twist

- 50 grams of fresh Spinach
- ½ avocado
- 6 chopped cubes of pineapple
- ½ teaspoon of cinnamon
- 1 cup of water

Blend this all together in a blender

Benefits:
Spinach consists of various important components that have been found to be promising in the prevention of various cancers. These examinations include bladder, prostate, liver and lung cancer. Different components in spinach such as folic acid, tocopherol and chlorophyllin work through different mechanisms to treat and protect cancer patients. There are studies that have shown that spinach is very effective against aggressive prostate cancer it is associated with epoxyxanthophyls, neoxanthin and violaxanthin that researchers say have a connection to directly reduce tumor activity and the spread of cancer throughout the body. (Rong Wang Department of Biochemistry and Food Science Toshio FURUMOTO Department of Biochemistry and Food Science Koichiro MOTOYAMA Department of Biochemistry and Food Science, Katsuichiro OKAZAKI of Life Sciences, Faculty of Agriculture, Kagawa University Akira KONDO Department of Biochemistry and Food Science Hiroshi FUKUI Department of Biochemistry and Food Science

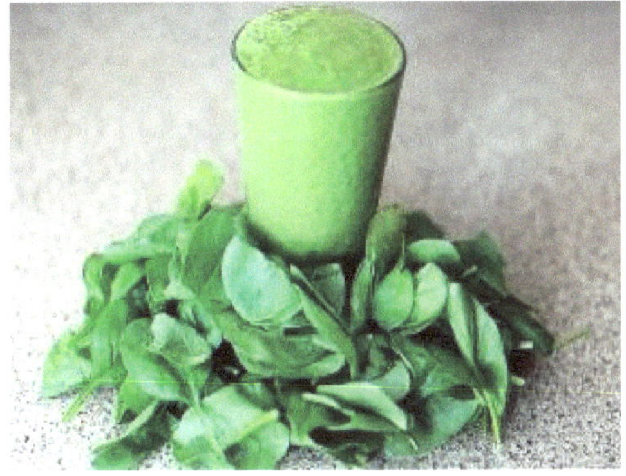

Benefits and facts about herbs and fruits.

We all grew up that our parents told us to eat fruit and vegetables, that it is healthy for you. But what do we really know about vegetables, fruit and herbs? Do we actually know what effect it has on our body and what benefits we all derive from it? There have been enough investigations in the medical field and are still ongoing, that it can even help and to combat certain diseases and health conditions. Fortunately, we are only getting wiser because the numbers that we are only getting older are not lying. We become more aware of what we eat and what resources we have at our disposal.

That is why I will list a number of herbs, vegetables and fruit here. Mainly those we use most in everyday life and / or should use if you didn't already. The knowledge it gives you is refreshing and believe me if you integrate them into your daily life you will be grateful to yourself in the future. Such small adjustments can do wonders in your life.

Let's start with the following herbs.

Ginger

Ginger is praised all over the world for its effect against nausea, vomiting, morning sickness and other digestive complaints, the smell of ginger is aromatic and it has a very distinct taste. This spice is delicious in many dishes, smoothies and juices. If you combine it with meat, the meat becomes more tender because it contains a protein-splitting enzyme.

Ginger has also been used in Asia for thousands of years because of its healing properties. It is a source of magnesium, potassium, vitamin B6 and powerful antioxidants. It is been used to heal among other things:

anti-inflammatory, heartburn, stomach ulcer, Humps, Cough Headache High Cholesterol Itching Toothache Stomach and intestinal disorders including irritable bowel syndrome, flatulence, bloating Menstrual problems Migraine (Morning) nausea Bursa and tendon inflammation Flu and cold Flatulence and burping (farmers)

(Source Wikipedia)

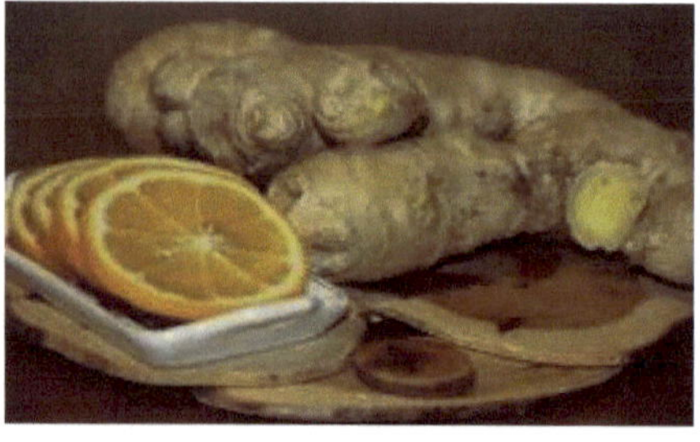

<u>**Celery**</u>

In a lot of research's, it is shown that celery has a positive influence on your cholesterol and on your overall health. Celery contains a unique substance called 3nbutylphtalide. This substance is known to lower the fat in your blood. In addition, celery, like asparagus, also contains a lot of potassium. This is an important mineral that is needed for nerve stimulation and maintaining normal blood pressure. Furthermore, potassium is necessary for the contraction of the muscles and for the energy management in the muscles. Potassium is also moisture-repellent

Celery contains antioxidants and polysaccharides that are known for their anti-inflammatory effect. Also, research has shown that celery has a positive effect on high blood pressure. This is because, among other things, celery contains the substance hexanoic acid that, among other things, stimulates blood circulation.

A 2010 study in the Journal of Pharmaceutical Biology, researchers concluded that celery contains a special type of ethanol extract that is useful in protecting the inside of the digestive tract to help against ulcers.

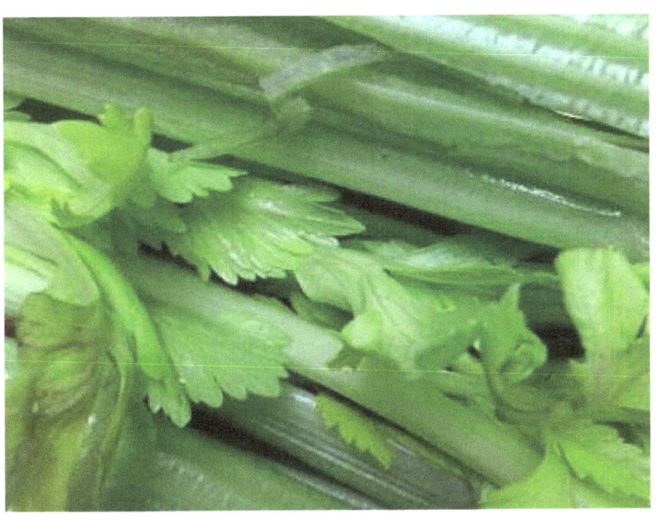

Mint

The use of mint goes back centuries to Ancient Egypt. According to the Ancient Greeks, mint was created by the jealousy of the god Hades. In the Middle Ages, the herb was already cultivated because of its medicinal properties.

Mint does not only ensure you a fresh breath, but dental hygiene in general. Mint has an antibacterial effect in combination with an anti-inflammatory effect. Mint is beneficial against toothache, abscesses, gum disease and other disorders.

The anti-inflammatory effect of mint also helps with muscle pain.

Mint is also recommended for stomach and intestinal problems. The Moroccans already drink this mint tea for century's because it helps against stomach cramps, flatulence, indigestion, bloating and diarrhea.

They also say it helps against colds; the antibacterial effect also fights the germs.

Besides al the healing effects it a delightful herb to extract tea from, drink your tea with honey or mix it with dinner recipes.

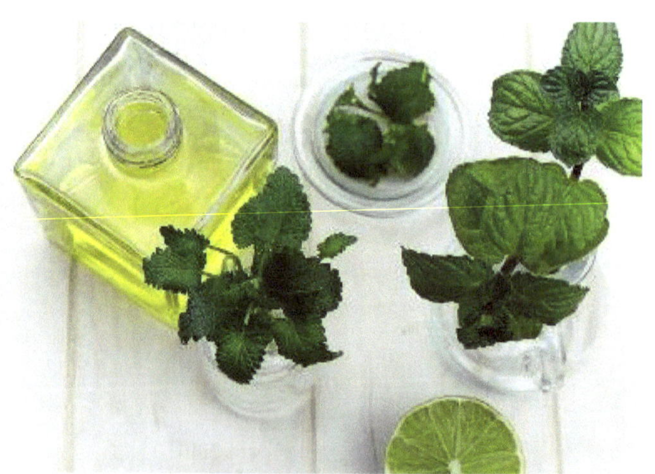

Pomegranate

Well what can I say about this super fruit there is too much to tell you about it that I would need a book only for the pomegranate and what benefits this super fruit has for you. But I will try to give you the top benefits of this fruit I will start with….

Fight cancer

A pomegranate has a high concentration of antioxidants. More than other fruits. Antioxidants ensure that the risk of cancer is reduced. Studies have shown that when people eat pomegranate on a regularly base, the risk of breast, lung and prostate cancer is clearly reduced. The pomegranates **can** cause that cancer cell development to be delayed in some, it contains a substance that prevents cancer from spreading.

Studies have also shown that it reduces blood flow to cancer cells. This causes the cancer cells to starve. This is published in 2008 in the International Journal of Oncology. In this study, mice received human prostate cancer cells. The mice were given a 4week cure with the pomegranate extract. The tumors became considerably smaller in the mice during that period. In addition, it is on 50 men who had tested prostate cancer. They drank one glass of fresh pomegranate juice a day. This fought the cancer in such a way that the need for chemotherapy greatly decreased. (source the International Journal of Oncology)

Protects your skin

A pomegranate contains antioxidants. This ensures that the damage caused by UV rays is reduced. They also counteract free radical and also stimulate the production of collagen.

Helps with erectile dysfunction

For the men pomegranate helps with erectile dysfunction.

The pomegranate also helps to a limited extent against erectile dysfunction. It is nice to know that you can also improve your erectile dysfunction with a natural remedy instead of a chemical.

It can help prevent acne

Acne is often caused by a hormonal imbalance or by digestive problems.

Eating pomegranate, can be remedied by combating the actual cause of acne. It resolves digestive problems and stimulates good circulation. The pomegranate contains a healthy amount of iron. Iron ensures that oxygen can be better absorbed into the blood. Oxygen is transported to the skin, making it look fresh and smooth again. It contains high level of vitamin C. This is an effective antioxidant that protects the skin against harmful free radicals Vitamin C also regulates the production of sebum. That is an oily release of the sebaceous glands to the skin. Too much sebum entering the skin, will cause you to get acne. Pomegranate also stimulates skin cell regeneration.

Reduces stress

In a study by Queen Margaret University in Edinburgh has shown that pomegranates can reduce stress. It causes the stress hormone cortisol in the saliva to decrease significantly by drinking the juice of a pomegranate. The people who participated in the study felt less stressed after drinking a glass of pomegranate juice.

Natural blood thinner

The seeds of a pomegranate contain a large number of antioxidants that act as blood thinners. This prevents platelets from coagulating and prevents the development of blood clots. it can prevent that people get clots in their hearts and veins, it helps preventing a heart attack or a stroke.

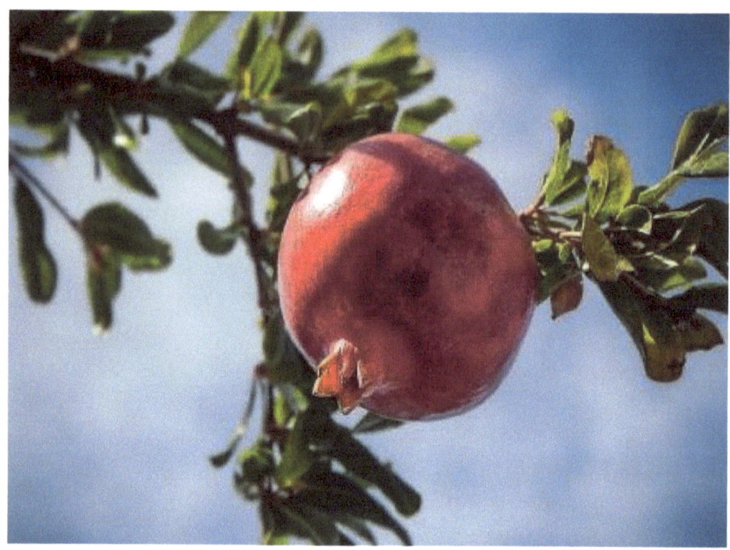

Avocados

Avocado have been and still are one of the most popular vegetables in the world. And of course, why would they not be when you know all their benefits that they bring to our health. You can make a diversity of recipes with it and it makes every dish just that little bit better.

Although avocados contain a lot of (healthy) fats, there are also quite a few benefits. We know for sure that the avocado will be here for a long time thanks to all these health benefits.

It is for your heart an avocado keeps the cardiologist at bay and away. Avocados are good for the health of your heart. Sandra J Arevalo, of the American Association of Diabetes Educators, says: "Healthy fats help to maintain a healthy cardiovascular system and reduce risk of stroke, heart attacks and other cardiovascular diseases."

Dietician Maureen Eyerman also agrees and says: "Monounsaturated fats found in avocados reduce LDL, or" bad "cholesterol levels, while increasing HDL," good "cholesterol levels."

Avocados also seem to contain good nutrients for your skin. The natural oils help your skin to hydrate and soften.

It helps against stress and other environmental factors. Antioxidants such as vitamins E and C also partly help keep your skin young you can find these vitamins in avocados.

It reduces stress Psychologist and nutrition expert Elise Museles says: "Magnesium helps you release tension and also sleep better. And when you're relaxed and well-rested, you're more likely reduce stress, Avocados contain these vitamins
It is also good for your hair and nails; avocados are also great for your hair and nails. The biotin contained in them nurture our hair and nails. In addition, vitamins B and E also protect your hair against dryness and hair loss.

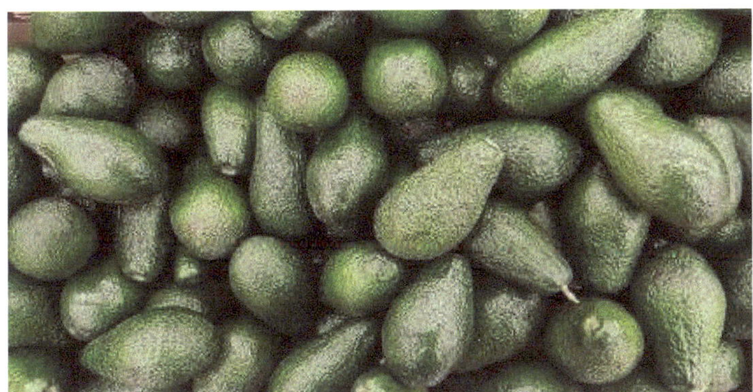

Conclusion word Detox

You have arrived at the end of Boost Your Fat Away Detox in 7-day program and I am sure a few pounds lighter than when you started 7 days ago. I assume after all the vitamin shakes and healthy minerals that you have consumed with the recipes from this book that you feel more energetic and better in your body. Your skin will also feel different and softer. And you will see the difference when you look in the mirror.

Apart from the external display, a lot has certainly changed on the inside. all waste is out of your body and your organs have been given a moment's rest to recover and clean up the toxins in your body.

Now it's a matter of redesigning your lifestyle in a healthy way and finding balance. A good continuation on the Boost your Fat Away in 7 days is my 21 @ diet Program.

If you want to find balance in your daily life or want to lose extra more weight, or you want to have nice day schedule recipes, then I highly recommend this. In the 21@ Diet Program is described all day menus with breakfast, snacks and dinner meals with recipes, including the calories that you take in on a daily bases and per each meal.

All in all, I hope that my program has helped you to take a step in the right direction, but if you have this book, I know that you are already working on it!

I wish you a healthy, enriching and balanced lifestyle.

Renee Anderson

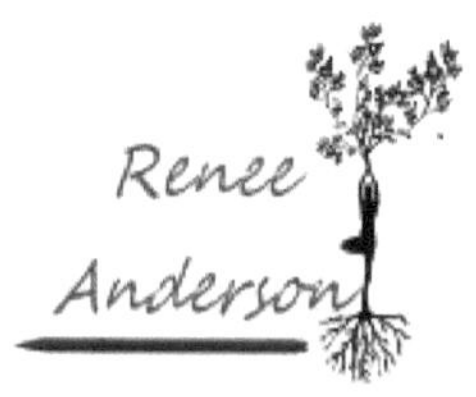